Arvinder Singh

Psoriatic Arthritis

Arvinder Singh

Psoriatic Arthritis
Conventional Radiology

LAP LAMBERT Academic Publishing

Impressum / Imprint

Bibliografische Information der Deutschen Nationalbibliothek: Die Deutsche Nationalbibliothek verzeichnet diese Publikation in der Deutschen Nationalbibliografie; detaillierte bibliografische Daten sind im Internet über http://dnb.d-nb.de abrufbar.

Alle in diesem Buch genannten Marken und Produktnamen unterliegen warenzeichen-, marken- oder patentrechtlichem Schutz bzw. sind Warenzeichen oder eingetragene Warenzeichen der jeweiligen Inhaber. Die Wiedergabe von Marken, Produktnamen, Gebrauchsnamen, Handelsnamen, Warenbezeichnungen u.s.w. in diesem Werk berechtigt auch ohne besondere Kennzeichnung nicht zu der Annahme, dass solche Namen im Sinne der Warenzeichen- und Markenschutzgesetzgebung als frei zu betrachten wären und daher von jedermann benutzt werden dürften.

Bibliographic information published by the Deutsche Nationalbibliothek: The Deutsche Nationalbibliothek lists this publication in the Deutsche Nationalbibliografie; detailed bibliographic data are available in the Internet at http://dnb.d-nb.de.

Any brand names and product names mentioned in this book are subject to trademark, brand or patent protection and are trademarks or registered trademarks of their respective holders. The use of brand names, product names, common names, trade names, product descriptions etc. even without a particular marking in this works is in no way to be construed to mean that such names may be regarded as unrestricted in respect of trademark and brand protection legislation and could thus be used by anyone.

Coverbild / Cover image: www.ingimage.com

Verlag / Publisher:
LAP LAMBERT Academic Publishing
ist ein Imprint der / is a trademark of
AV Akademikerverlag GmbH & Co. KG
Heinrich-Böcking-Str. 6-8, 66121 Saarbrücken, Deutschland / Germany
Email: info@lap-publishing.com

Herstellung: siehe letzte Seite /
Printed at: see last page
ISBN: 978-3-659-43136-4

Copyright © 2013 AV Akademikerverlag GmbH & Co. KG
Alle Rechte vorbehalten. / All rights reserved. Saarbrücken 2013

ACKNOWLEDGEMENT

Dedicated to the Universal light, the God, who guided me through whole of the way in my research work.

Regards to my respected teacher and mentor, Dr.Sudesh Khanna and my guide Dr.S.P.Dewan for their great efforts for supervising and leading me to accomplish this fine work.

Words falls short for the support and guidance given by my wife, Dr Manjeet Kaur. And love and affection given by my daughter Simrita and sons Anshu and Amitoj.

To my friends and colleagues who were source of kind support and encouragement.

Above all my gratitude to all the patients who gave their confidence and trust in me to compile and complete my research work with all their support to me.

I thank them all with my deepest gratitude, love and affection.

TABLE OF CONTENTS

SR.NO.	CHAPTER	PAGE NO.
1.	INTRODUCTION	1-7
2.	OBJECTIVES	8
3.	MATERIAL & METHODS	9-10
4.	OBSERVATIONS	11-25
5.	DISCUSSION	26-41
6.	SUMMARY & CONCLUSIONS	42-43
7.	COMMENTS	44
8.	REFERENCES	45-47

CHAPTER I

INTRODUCTION

Psoriasis is a common, genetically determined disease of skin consisting of well defined pink or dull red lesions with characteristic silver scales over them. It affects 1-2% of the population.

Psoriatic arthritis may be defined as an inflammatory disease of joints in patients with cutaneous psoriasis with or without nail changes and with a negative serological test for rheumatoid arthritis. The incidence of arthritis in patients with cutaneous psoriasis is about 6-7%.

There is strong relationship between generalized pustular psoriasis, erythrodermic psoriasis and arthritis. Also there is strong genetic predisposition and HLA-B27 association in psoriatic arthritis especially spondylitic form. Trauma may also play a role in induction of psoriasis and arthritis.

Nail changes, onchylosis, nail pitting are especially associated with involvement of distal interphalangeal joint and terminal tuft resorption. There is a slight male predominance in psoriatic arthritis with male to female ratio 1.29:1.

Alibert in 1822, was first to recognize the occurrence of joint changes in psoriasis. Bazin in 1860, named cases of psoriasis with joint changes as psoriatic arthritis, and the cases of psoriasis without joint changes were named as psoriasis herpetica. Bourdilion in 1888, published his masterly thesis on "psoriasis et arthropathies" describing psoriasis as a separate entity. However lack of radiological evidence was there.

Garrod and Geoffrey[1] studied three cases of psoriasis with arthritis. Due to presence of radiological evidence they concluded that psoriasis with arthritis is a definite clinical entity.

Mackenna[2] in a "refresher course for general practitioners, the problems of psoriasis" quoted that arthropathic psoriasis usually begins with involvement of joints of distal phalanges of hands and feet. Sherman[3] observed the clinical and radiological findings in 7 cases of psoriasis with joints involvement. The earliest changes were seen in interphalangeal joints, consisting of marginal erosions i.e. bare area erosions at the very edges of the phalanges.

Eisenstadt et al[4] studied a case of psoriasis with arthritis mutilans, and revealed that arthritis mutilans is a common entity and named it as "Arthritis Psoriatica".

Wright et al[5] studied the radiographic appearances of psoriasis with arthritis in 39 patients, 32 with erosive arthritis, 6 with degenerative changes and 1 with gout. Radiographs of hands, feet and sacroiliac joints were taken routinely. It was noted that erosions with little or no osteoporosis was found in psoriatic arthritis than in those with rheumatoid arthritis. He commented that psoriasis has predilection for distal interphalangeal joint in 52% cases. The changes were erosions, loss of cartilage, expansion of bases of terminal phalynx, sometimes with mild flexion deformity and rarely bony ankylosis.

Wright et al[6] studied 154 patients of psoriasis with arthritis and suggested that psoriasis has negative Rose Waaler sheep cell agglutination test i.e. rheumatoid factor. There is predilection for distal joints of hands and feet and unlike other arthritides it commonly began in distal interphalangeal joints. The arthritis was more often asymmetrical than in rheumatoid arthritis.

Avila et al[7] studied 150 patients of psoriasis with arthritis and observed five radiological signs as follow:-

- Destructive arthritis involving predominately distal and proximal interphalangeal joints of hands and feet.
- Abnormally widened joint spaces in some cases.
- Bony ankylosis of the affected joints.
- Resorption of tufts of distal phalanges of hands and feet.
- Bone proliferation at the bases of distal phalanges especially great toes.

Baker et al[8] studied 60 patients and revealed on x rays the involved joints. Predominantly terminal interphalangeal joints (8cases), whittling of terminal phalanx(5 cases), interphalangeal joint arthritis of hallux(10cases).28% had features of sacroiliitis.

Peterson et al[9] studied 39 cases of psoriasis and 32 cases of Reiter's disease. They found out that destruction and deformity of joints was more frequent in psoriatic arthritis, while in Reiter's disease joint destruction was less common. Also in Reiter's disease urethritis is invariably present. Both conditions show features of sacroiliac joint involvement with negative rheumatoid factor.

Miller et al[10] studied a case of psoriatic arthritis with extensive distal interphalangeal resorption. There is whittling away of bone in distal phalanges giving 'peg shaped' appearance characteristic of psoriatic arthritis.

Kate Killebrew[11] studied the radiographic findings of psoriatic spondylitis in 21 patients. Following findings were noted in spine.

- Coarse asymmetrical non marginal syndesomphyte formation, commonly seen in the thoracolumbar region.

- High incidence of sacroiliitis.

Martel et al[13] reviewed 50 patients of psoriatic arthritis and 34 patients of erosive arthritis, and suggested that patients with psoriasis had negative rheumatoid factor.

Oriente et al[14] 1984 studied 184 patients of psoriasis. Arthritis was seen in 62(34.4%) cases and polyarticular form was common. Arthritis mutilans was seen in 2.3% cases and spondylitis and/or sacroiliitis in 20.9% cases. Nail changes were seen in 63% cases. Male to female ratio was 1:1. Skin lesions preceded arthritis in 64.5% cases and in 19.3% arthritis antedated psoriasis and in 16.2% cases psoriasis and arthritis started simultaneously.

Rajindra et al[15] studied seronegative arthropathies of foot. They concluded that 5-10% of patients with cutaneous psoriasis developed arthritis. Men were more commonly involved. Nail changes were commonly associated. In foot, interphalangeal joint of great toe was involved in form of bare area erosions. Periosteitis occurs in shafts of metatarsals and phalanges. Widening of joint space occurred latter in disease due to deposition of fibrous tissue. Tapering and resorption of terminal phalanges of toes together with nail changes are highly suggestive of psoriatic arthropathy.

El-Khoury at al[16] studied the seronegative spondyloarthopathies. He found that spondylitis was seen in 20-30% cases of psoriasis. The syndesmophytes seen in psoriatic arthritis were indistinguishable from Reiter's disease, and history of urethritis was invariably seen in the latter.

M Backhaus at al[17] studied arthritis of the finger joints in 60 patients. They found that MRI, ultrasound, and 3-phase bone scintigraphy are more sensitive than conventional radiography in detecting inflammatory joint processes. Scintigraphy, however appears to be of limited value because of its lack of specificity. Ultrasound allows a sensitive detection of the inflammatory soft tissue process in the form of synovitis and tenosynovitis, but is not optimal for the detection of erosions. MRI is more sensitive than conventional radiography in detecting both inflammatory signs and erosions. A major drawback of MRI is the expensive imaging procedure,especially when using contrast agents. MRI and ultrasound are valuable diagnostic modalities for patients with suspected arthritis who have normal radiologic findings.

Marsal et al[18] studied 73 patients for clinical, radiographic and HLA associations as markers for different patterns of psoriatic arthritis. They studied that the erosive disease was independent of duration of disease.

Brockbank et al[19] wrote about the diagnosis and management of psoriatic arthritis. Treating the skin alone seems to have little impact on joint disease, and the relationship between skin and joints is still unclear. It is now recognized that PsA can be a destructive arthritis with an increased morbidity and mortality. Anti-tumor necrosis factor agents, such as etanercept and infliximab, have shown considerable significant clinical benefit and provided the hope.

Gladman et al[20] studied epidemiology, clinical features, course and outcome of psoriatic arthritis. PsA typically presents as an oligoarticular and mild disease. However, with time PsA becomes polyarticular, and it is a severe disease in at least 20% of patients. Patients with PsA who present with polyarticular disease are at risk for disease progression. In addition to progression of clinical and radiological damage, health related quality of life is reduced among patients with PsA.

PA Ory et al[21] published a report on psoriatic arthritis and imaging.They suggested that traditionally, joint damage has been recorded using plain radiographs. Characteristic radiographic features of PsA include joint erosions, joint space narrowing, bony proliferation including periarticular and shaft periosteitis, osteolysis including "pencil in cup" deformity and acro-osteolysis, ankylosis, spur formation, and spondylitis. New imaging modalities, including ultrasound, bone scanning, and magnetic resonance imaging may help in both diagnosis and follow up of patients with PsA.

CP Rajendran et al[22] studied 116 patients of psoriatic arthritis. Out of theses 78 were males, 38 were females with male to female ratio 2:1. Peak incidence (69%) was in the fourth and fifth decades. One patient had juvenile psoriatic arthritis (onset <16 years of age).Symmetric polyarthritis (48.3%) was the commonest subtype. Arthritis followed the skin lesions in 50.8% of patients, preceded in 12.1% and occurred simultaneously in 37.1%. Extra-articular features like sausage digits (19%), enthesitis (7.8%) and eye manifestations (1.7%) like conjunctivitis and uveitis were observed. Psoriasis vulgaris (81%) was the commonest psoriatic lesion. Scalp (57.8%) was the most common hidden site. All the three patients with DIP arthritis alone had nail lesions. ESR and C-reactive protein were elevated in 51.7% and 43.9% of patients respectively. Radiographic features like sacroiliitis (11.2%), calcaneal spur (7.8%), erosions (5.2%) and syndesmophytes (5.2%) were observed. One patient had 'pencil-in-cup deformity'.

Kane et al[23] studied 129 patients of psoriatic arthritis and found that mean age was 40.4 years, mean age of duration of disease was 9.9 months, nail dystrophy was seen in 675 cases,39% patients had DIPJ involvement.

CHAPTER II

OBJECTIVES

1. To determine radiologically, various skeletal changes in clinically diagnosed cases of psoriasis with arthritis.

2. To study the distribution pattern of various skeletal changes seen in psoriasis associated with commonly involved joints.

MATERIAL AND METHODS

Thirty three clinically diagnosed cases of psoriasis with arthritis irrespective of age, sex, duration and extent of disease were selected at random from department of dermatology and STD, Government Medical College and Hospital, Amritsar. All the cases were tested for rheumatoid factor and only seronegative patients were included in the study. Finally out of 33 psoriatic arthritis study cases, 30 were included in the present study. The remaining three cases were excluded because they were seropositive for rheumatoid factor. A detailed history in each case indicating the extent, activity and duration of disease, including personal and family history, physical examination of skin lesions and clinically involved joints were recorded on special proforma.

Laboratory Investigations: cases selected were put to following laboratory investigations:-

1. Hemoglobin: Hemoglobin of all the patients was tested by haemoglobinometer.

2. Erythrocytic sedimentation rate: Early fasting sample of blood was taken and erythrocytic sedimentation rate was recorded in mm 1st hour by Western Green method.

3. Rheumatoid factor: Each patient was tested for this serological test. All the patients who were seronegative for rheumatoid factor were included in the study. All seropositive patients were excluded.

4. Radiological Examination:

Each patient was X Rayed for following joints:-

i) X ray both hands – AP view

ii) X ray both feet – AP view

iii) X ray dorsolumbar spine – AP view

iv) X ray both sacroiliac joints - AP view

CHAPTER III

OBSERVATIONS

The results of the present study were compiled in tabulated form and discussed as follows:-

TABLE I

AGE DISTRIBUTION IN 30 STUDY CASES

Age in years	Number			Percentage
	Male	Female	Total	
20-30	-	2	2	6.6
31-40	5	2	7	23.3
41-50	8	5	13	43.5
51-60	4	2	6	20.0
61-70	2	-	2	6.6

The age range was between 28-70years with average age of about 49 years. The maximum number of cases were 26(86.6%) cases were between age 31-60 years.

TABLE II

SEX DISTRIBUTION IN 30 STUDY CASES

Sex	Number of cases	Percentage
Male	19	63.0
Female	11	37.0

There were 19(63%) male cases and 11(37%) female cases, with male to female ratio 1.72:1.

TABLE III

DURATION OF SKIN LESIONS IN 30 STUDY CASES

Duration of illness	No. of cases		Total(%age)
	Male	Female	
<6 months	1	-	1(3.3)
6 months-2 years	-	1	1(3.3)
2-5 years	4	7	11(36.6)
>5 years	14	3	17(56.8)

Most of the cases i.e. 17(56.8%) had history of skin lesions for more than 5 years, followed by 11(36.6%) cases with history of 2-5years.The remaining 2(6.6%) cases had duration of illness less than 2 years. The minimum duration of illness was 3 months and one case had history maximum of 25 years.

TABLE IV

DURATION OF ARTHRITIS IN 30 STUDY CASES

Duration of illness	No. of cases		Total(%age)
	Male	Female	
<6 months	2	1	3(10.0)
6 months-2 years	6	4	10(33.3)
2-5 years	6	3	9(30.0)
>5 years	5	3	8(26.7)

The maximum no. of 10(33.3%)cases had duration of arthritis between 6 months to 2years, 9(30%) cases between 2 to 5years.8(26.7%) were having duration of illness more than 5 years followed by 3(10%)cases with illness of less than 6 months.The minimum duration of illness was 3 months in 1 case and maximum of 20years in another case.

TABLE V

ONSET OF SKIN LEASIONS AND ARTHRITIS IN 30 STUDY CASES

Onset of arthritis	No. of cases			Percentage
	Male	Female	Total	
Skin lesions preceded arthritis	14	10	24	80.0
Skin lesions concomitant with arthritis	5	1	6	20.0

The above table shows that in 24(80%) cases skin lesions preceded arthritis, while in 6(20%) cases skin lesions started concomitantly.

TABLE VI

FAMILY HISTORY RELEVENCE IN 30 STUDY CASES

	No.of cases			Percentage
	Male	Female	Total	
Family history	3	2	5	16.5

The above table shows that there were only 5(16.5%) patients with positive family history and remaining 25(83.5%) had no relevant family history.

TABLE VII

LABORATORY INVESTIGATIONS IN 30 STUDY CASES

Investigations	No.of cases			Percentage
	Male	Female	Total	
Hemoglobin <10gm% >10gm%	5 14	4 7	9 21	30.0 70.0
ESR(Wester-green method) <20mm 1st Hour >20mm 1st Hour	3 16	1 10	4 26	13.2 85.8

There were 9(30%) cases who suffered from mild anemia in whom the estimated hemoglobin was less that 10gm%. ESR was raised in 26(85.8%) cases.

TABLE VIII

CLINICAL PATTERN OF PSORIASIS IN 30 STUDY CASES

Clinical pattern	No. of cases			Percentage
	Male	Female	Total	
Discoid psoriasis	13	7	20	66.0
Erythrodermic psoriasis	2	1	3	10.0
Psoriasis of hands	2	1	3	10.0
Psoriasis of feet	1	1	2	6.6
Psoriasis of hands and feet	1	1	2	6.6

The maximum no. of cases 20(66%) were having discoid psoriasis, followed by 3(10.0%)cases of erythrodermic psoriasis and 3(6.6%)cases of psoriasis of hands only. Psoriasis of feet only and hands and feet were seen in 2(6.6%)cases each.

TABLE IX

CLINICAL PATTERN OF PSORIATIC ARTHRITIS IN 30 STUDY CASES

Clinical pattern	No. of cases			Percentage
	Male	Female	Total	
Pain only	11	7	18	60.0
Pain & swelling	4	1	5	16.6
Pain, swelling & mild deformity	1	3	4	13.4
Gross deformity only	3	-	3	10.0

The commonest pattern of arthritis was pain only in 18(60%) cases followed by pain and swelling in 5(16.6%) cases. Pain, swelling and mild deformity in 4(13.4%) cases. Gross deformity was seen in 3(10%) cases.

TABLE X

ASSOCIATED NAIL CHANGES IN 30 STUDY CASES

Nail changes	No.of cases			Percentage
	Male	Female	Total	
Present	16	8	24	80.0
Absent	4	2	6	20.0

24(80%) cases showed various nail changes in form of pitting, nail plate thickening, subungual keratosis and onchylosis. The remaining 6(20%) cases did not show any type of nail changes.

TABLE XI

BONY INVOLVEMENT IN 30 STUDY CASES

Parts involved	No. of cases			Percentage
	Male	Female	Total	
Hands	13	8	21	70.0
Feet	13	6	19	63.3
Dorsolumbar spine	6	4	10	33.0
Sacroiliac joints	7	3	10	33.0

The most commonly affected part in psoriatic arthritis was hands in 21(70%) cases. Feet were involved in 19(63.3%)cases, dorsolumbar spine in 10(33%)cases and sacroiliac joints in10(33%)cases.

TABLE XII

PATTERN OF BONY INVOLVEMENT IN 30 STUDY CASES

Clinical pattern	No.of cases			Percentage
	Male	Female	Total	
Hands only	3	2	5	16.5
Feet only	2	1	3	10.0
SI joints	2	-	2	6.6
DL spine	1	-	1	3.3
Hands and feet	4	3	7	23.1
Hands,feet,SI joints,DL spine	2	2	4	13.2
Hands,feet,SI joints	2	-	2	6.6
Feet and DL spine	1	1	2	6.6
DL spine and SI joints	-	1	1	63.3
Hands and SI	-	1	1	3.3

joints				
Hands and DL spine	-	1	1	3.3
Hands, feet and DL spine	1	-	1	3.3

The maximum no. of cases 7(23.1%) showed involvement of both hands and feet, 5(16.5%) cases showed involvement of hands only and 3(10%) cases showed involvement of feet only. In 4(13.2%) cases hands, feet, SI joints and DL spine were involved.

TABLE XIII

DISTRIBUTION OF RADIOLOGICAL FEATURES IN HANDS IN 30 STUDY CASES

Radiological features	No. of cases			Percentage
	Male	Female	Total	
Erosions at DIPJ	13	8	21	70.0
Tuft resorption	6	3	9	30.0
New bone formation	4	1	5	16.6
Loss of articular cartilage	3	1	4	13.3
Mild flexion deformity	1	3	4	13.3
Bony ankylosis	2	1	3	10.0

The commonest lesion observed in hands was erosions in 21(70%) cases. The erosions were most common in the bare areas of distal phalanges or around distal interphalangeal joints. The other radiological features were terminal tuft resorption 9(30%) cases, new bone formation at bases of terminal phalanges in 5(16.5%), mild flexion deformity in 4(13.3%) cases, loss of articular cartilage in 4(13.3%) cases and bony ankylosis in 3 (10%) cases.

TABLE XIV

RADIOLOGICAL FEATURES IN FEET IN 30 STUDY CASES

Radiological features	No. of cases			Percentage
	Male	Female	Total	
Erosions at DIPJ	13	6	19	63.4
Tuft resorption	2	5	7	23.0
New bone formation	5	1	6	20.0
Loss of articular cartilage	2	1	3	10.0
Mild flexion deformity	2	-	2	6.6
Bony ankylosis	1	1	1	3.3

In feet, the most common finding was new bone formation at the base of terminal phalanx of great toe in 19(63.4%) cases. It was followed by bare area erosions in 7(23%) cases, terminal tuft resorption in distal phalanges in 6(20%)cases, mild flexion deformity in 3(10%)cases, loss of articular cartilage 2(6.6%)cases and bony ankylosis 1(3.3%)case.

TABLE XV

DISTRIBUTION OF RADIOLOGICAL FEATURES IN DORSOLUMBAR SPINE

Radiological features	No. of cases			Percentage
	Male	Female	Total	
Syndesmophytes formation	6	4	10	33.0
Ankylosis	-	-	-	-

The only radiological finding was coarse, floating osteophytes and asymmetrical syndesmophytes formation in 10(33%) cases. No case of bony ankylosis was seen in DL spine.

TABLE XVI

RADIOLOGICAL FEATURES IN SACRIILIAC JOINTS IN 30 STUDY CASES

Radiological features	No. of cases			Percentage
	Male	Female	Total	
Articular erosions	6	1	7	23.0
Juxta-articular sclerosis	3	2	5	16.5
Ankylosis	2	-	2	6.6

The most common lesion observed in sacroiliac joints was articular erosions in 7(23%) cases, juxta articular sclerosis in 5(16.5%)cases and bony ankylosis was seen in 2(6.6%)cases only.

CHAPTER IV

DISCUSSION

Psoriasis is a common, genetically determined disease of skin constituted of well-defined pink or dull red lesions with characteristic silvery scaling (Figure -1). It affects 1-2% of population. Psoriatic arthritis may be defined as inflammatory disease of joints in a patient of psoriasis with a negative serological test for rheumatoid factor. Its incidence is about 6-7%of psoriatic patients.

Alibert in 1822 first recognized the occurrence of joint lesions in psoriasis. Bazin had named psoriatic arthritis to those cases of psoriasis that had joint lesions and the cases and the cases of psoriasis without joint lesions were named as psoriatic herpetica.

Garrod and Geoffrey[1] in 1924 studied three cases of psoriasis associated with arthritis. He concluded that the psoriasis with arthritis as a clinical entity and neither lesion can be regarded as a mere complication of the other.

Mackenna[2] in a "refresher course for general practitioner, the problem of psoriasis" quoted that arthropathic psoriasis usually begins with involvement of the joints of the terminal phalanges.

Sherman[3], Wright et al[5], Baker et al[8] were the main series of studies which have done maximum work for the study of psoriatic arthritis.

Camp et al[25] in text book of dermatology edited by cook et al has mentioned the radiological features as:-

- Distal interphalangeal joint involvement with erosion and expansion of the base of the terminal phalanx.

- Terminal tuft erosion of hand and feet.

- Arthritis mutilans giving 'pencil in cup' appearance.

- Oligoarthritis

- Sacroiliitis

- Spinal involvement-syndesmophyte may be present without sacroiliitis.

The present study was undertaken to determine radiologically, various skeletal changes in clinically diagnosed cases of psoriasis with arthritis and to study the distribution pattern of various skeletal changes seen in psoriasis associated with commonly involved joints. It was done in the Department of Radiodiagnosis cases referred from Skin & STD of Guru Nanak Dev Hospital /Government medical College, Amritsar. The study was conducted on 33 patients of psoriasis with arthritis based on clinical features. A detailed medical history along with complete cutaneous, physical and systemic examination and laboratory investigation was done in all of them. Finally 30 psoriatic cases with arthritis were enrolled in the present study and the remaining 3 cases that were positive for rheumatoid factor were excluded from the study.

Further investigations (Hb and ESR) and x ray examination was done in all the 30 cases.

The results of the study were compiled in a tabulated chart and compared with those reported in the literature.

AGE DISTRIBUTION

In our study, the maximum no. of cases i.e. 26(86.8%) were in the age group between 31-60years. However the minimum age of the patient suffering from this disease was 28 years and maximum age was 70 years. The average age was 49 years. The age groups which suffered least were between 20-30years and 61-71years.

CP Rajendran et al[22] conducted study on 116 patients with peak incidence of psoriatic arthritis was 69% in age group of 40-50years. The mean age was 40.9 years. Oriente et al[14] conducted study on 182 patients of psoriasis with arthritis and concluded that maximum age group affected was 40 to 60 years and the average age was 54.3years. So our study is consistent with the studies of CP Rajendran et al[22] and Oriente et al[14] to some extent.

SEX DISTRIBUTION

In our study the no.of males affected were 19(63%) and females were 11(37%). This showed male predominance. The male to female ratio was 1.72:1.

TABLE XVII

Author	Male	Female	Ratio
Wright et al[5]	18	16	1.13:1
Avila et al[7]	28	22	1.29:1
CP Rajendran et al[22]	78	38	2:1

| Present study | 19 | 11 | 1.72:1 |

The above table shows different studies. All these studies show findings of male predominance which are consistent with our study.

DURATION OF SKIN LESIONS

Maximum no. of cases i.e. 17(56.1%) had history of skin lesions for more than 5 years. It was followed by 11(36.6%) cases who had history of skin lesion for 2-5years, 2(6.6%) cases had duration of illness less than 2 years. Our findings of duration of skin lesions are consistent with Oriente et al[14] who in their study of 182 cases reported similar findings.

DURATION OF ARTHRITIS

Maximum no. of cases i.e.10(33%) had duration of arthritis between 6 months to 2 years followed by 9(30%)cases between 2-5 years. 8(26.4%)cases had duration of illness more than 5 years followed by 3(10%) cases with duration of illness less than 6 months. The range of duration of arthritis in our study was 6months to 20years. Avila et al[7] studied 150 cases and reported that the duration of arthritis ranged from 1month to 46years whereas Martel et al[13] had reported a range of duration of arthritis from 2-36 years in their 50 study cases. Both the studies are at variance with our study.

ONSET OF SKIN LESIONS AND ARTHRITIS

In our study the skin lesions preceded arthritis in 24(80%) cases while skin lesions concomitantly in 6(20%) cases. Kate Killebrew et al[11] studied 87 cases and reported that the skin lesions preceded arthritis in 43% cases and skin lesions appeared concomitantly with arthritis in 195cases. CP Rajendran et al[22] conducted study on 116 patients and reported that arthritis followed the skin lesions in 50.8% of patients, preceded in 12.1% and occurred simultaneously in 37.1%. Our findings of skin lesions preceded arthritis are in agreement with above mentioned studies.

FAMILY HISTORY

Family history was positive in 5(16.5%) cases in our study. Baker et al[8] reported 10% parental manifestation in their study of 60 patients in pure dominant pattern of inheritance that 50% patients would be affected.

LABORATORY INVESTIGATIONS

Following laboratory investigations were done on every patient.

1. *Hemoglobin:* The lowest level of hemoglobin measures in patients was 8.0gm% and highest was 14.2% with average of 10.8%. The level of hemoglobin was normal in 21(70%) patients and it was abnormal(less than 10gm%) in 9 patients i.e 30% of patients and so they suffered from mild anemia. Baker et al[8] studied 60 patients and noticed anemia in 32% of cases. This is consistent with our study.

2. *Erythrocyte sedimentation rate:* In our study the ESR of the patients was between 12-60mm with the average 36mm in 1st hour by Western Green method. Only 4 patients in our study were having normal ESR(less than 20mm 1st hour).

Our observations of increased study ESR were in agreement with the findings of Baker et al[8] who in their study of 60 cases also found raised ESR in 70% cases. CP Rajendran et al[22] in their study of 116 patients found raised ESR in 51% cases.

CLINICAL PATTERN OF PSORIASIS

The commonest clinical patterns of psoriasis observed was discoid psoriasis i.e. 20 (66%) cases (Figure-1a). Other patterns were erythrodermic psoriasis (Figure-1b) i.e. 3(10%) cases, psoriasis of hands only 3(10%) cases(Figure-1c,d) and psoriasis of feet only 2(6.6%) cases.

CLINICAL PATTERNS OF PSORIATIC ARTHRITIS

Commonest clinical presentation of arthritis was pain only 10(60%) cases. Other presentations were pain and swelling in 5(16%) cases, pain, swelling and mild deformity in 4(13.3%) cases and gross deformity in 3(10%) cases.

Kate killebrew[11] reported pain in 85.55cases of their 87study cases. Wright et al[5] reported mild deformity in 19% of their 154 study cases. Martel et al[13] reported mild deformity in 18% and gross deformity in 10% cases in their 50 study cases.

NAIL CHANGES

Nail changes were observed in 24(80%) cases in form of pitting, nail plate thickening, subungual keratosis and onchylosis(Figure.1d).

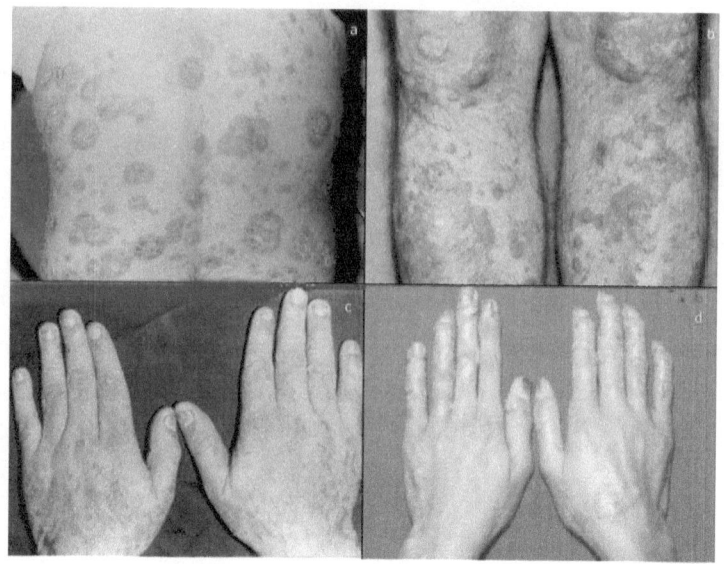

Figure.1-Photograph (a)showing scaly erythematous maculopapular lesion at the back of the patient suggestive of discoid type of psoriasis.(b)showing dull red eczematous, psoriatic lesions on both legs(c)showing dull red papular psoriatic skin lesions on both hands(d) showing eczematous psoriatic skin lesions on hands with nails changes.

Oriente et al[14] reported nail changes in 62% of their 182 study cases.Camp[25] reported nail changes in 75% cases in their study. El Khoury et al[16] reported nail changes in 80% of their 52 study cases. The results of all of above are in consistent with our findings. CP Rajendran et al[22] in their 116 study cases found nail changes in 30.2% cases.J E Brockbank et al[24] reported nail changes in 80% of 240 study cases.

BONY INVOLVEMENT

Bony involvement was seen maximum in hands i.e.21(70%) cases followed by feet 19(63.3%) cases, dorsolumbar spine and sacroiliac joints in 10(33%)cases.

Martel et al[13] reported involvement of hands and feet in 96% and 80% respectively in their series of 50 study cases. The above study reveals that maximum bony involvement was seen in hands and feet.

Kate killebrew[11] have reported involvement of dorsolumbar spine in 10-36% cases. Their findings are almost similar to our findings of involvement of dorsolumbar spine in our study.

Peterson et al[9] observed involvement of sacroiliac joints in 36% of their 39 study cases. The results of their study are compatible with our study.

PATTERN OF BONY INVOLVEMENT

The maximum no. of cases 7(23.1%) showed involvement of hands and feet only. In 4(13.2%) cases hands, feet, SI joints and DL spine were involved.

Rajendra et al[15] reported involvement of hands and feet in 50% of their 42 study cases. So their results are at variance with our study.

DISTRIBUTION OF RADIOLOGICAL FEATURES IN HANDS

Commonest radiological findings observed in hands were erosions at bare areas of DIPJ in 21(70%) cases (Figure-2a,b).

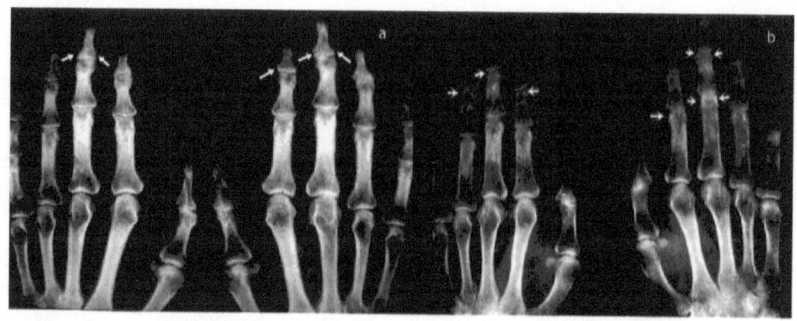

Figure.2 (a)X ray both hands AP view showing bare area erosions at the bases of distal phalanges (white arrows) with evidence of tuft resorption (b)X ray both hands AP views showing bare area erosions at distal phalanges and proximal interphalangeal joints (white arrows).No evidence of tuft resorption.

Other radiological findings were terminal tuft resorption 9(30%)cases(Figure.3), new bone formation at bases of terminal phalanges in 5(16.5%) cases, mild flexion deformity in 4(13.3%) cases and bony ankylosis in 3(10%)cases (Figure.4).

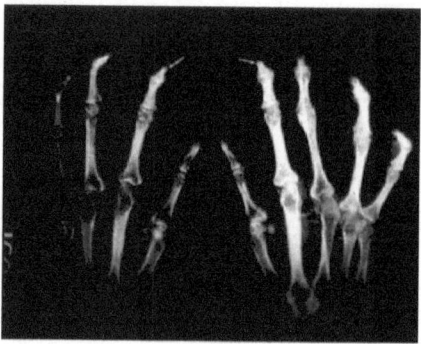

Figure.3- X ray both hands AP view showing mild flexion deformities at distal interphalangeal joints with tuft resorption.

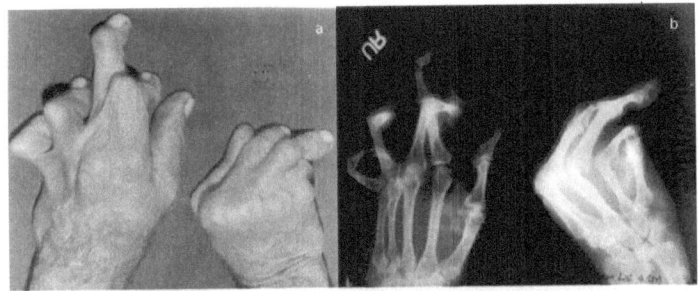

Figure.4-(a)Photograph showing marked deformities in both hands(b)X rays both hands AP view of same patients showing gross flexion and extension deformities at DIPJ, PIPJ and metacarpophalangeal joints-Arthritis Mutilans.

Schumacher et al[12] also observed similar evidence of erosions in hand in 76% of 22 study cases. D Kane et al[23] observed erosions in hands in 32(27%) of 129 study cases. This is at variance with our study.

Peterson et al[9] noted tuft resorption in 22% of their 39 study cases which is slightly less than in our study.

Wright et al[6] reported new bone formation at bases of terminal phalanges of hands and feet both in 35% of 154 study cases, thus our results could not be correlated with their study.

Martel et al[13] noticed mild flexion deformity due to loss of articular cartilage in 18% of their 50 study cases. Their results are slightly on higher side.

Wright et al[6] reviewed 154 cases and got bony ankylosis in 16% cases whereas Peterson et al[9] got bony ankylosis in 5% of 39 study cases. Both these studies regarding bony ankylosis are at variance with our study.

DISTRIBUTION OF RADIOLOGICAL FEATURES IN FEET

Commonest radiological finding observed in feet was new bone formation in 19(63.4%) cases at the bases of distal phalanx of great toe (Figure.5).

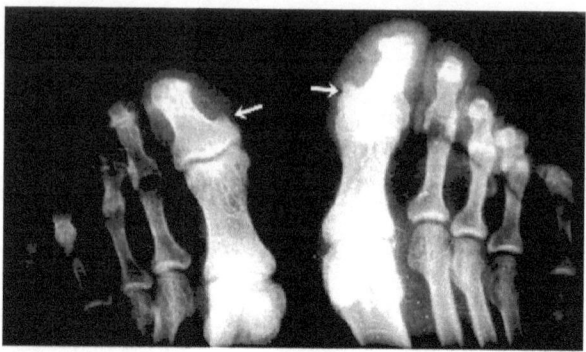

Figure.5 - X ray both feet AP views showing new bone formation on medial aspect of bases of both great toes (long arrow).

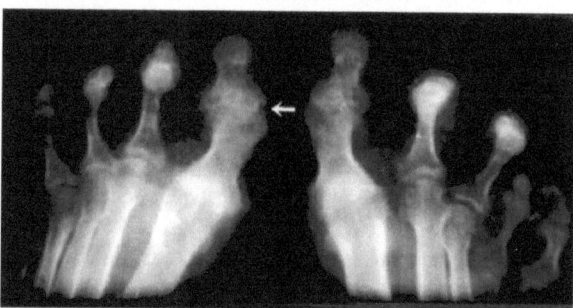

Figure.6 - X ray both feet AP views showing bare area erosions at the base of distal phalanx great toe right side with reduction of DIPJ space (white arrow). Broadening of bases of distal phalanges of both great toe are also seen.

Other radiological findings were erosions in the bare area of DIPJ in 7(23%) cases (Figure.6), 3(10%) cases tuft resorption (Figure.7), loss of articular cartilage in 2(6.6%) cases and bony ankylosis in 1(3.3%) cases (Figure.8).

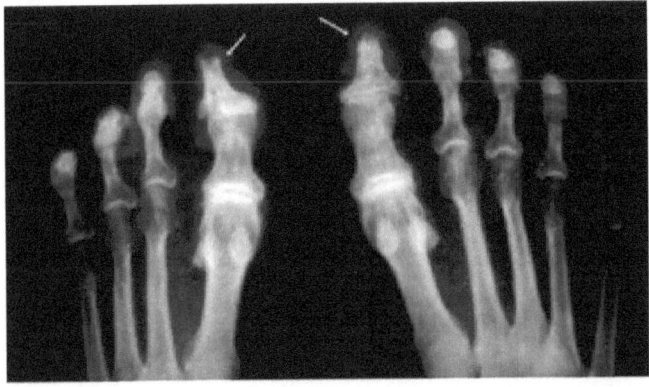

Figure.7- X rays both feet AP views showing tuft resorption of great toes (white arrows).

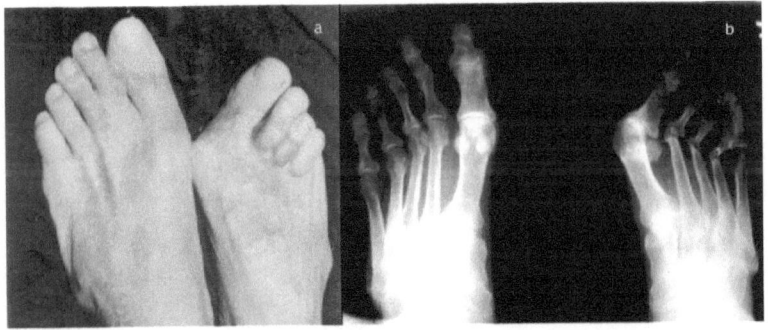

Figure.8-(a)Photograph showing marked asymmetric deformities in right foot(b)X rays both feet AP views of same patients showing gross deformities metatarsophalangeal joints of left foot with 'pencil in cup' appearance-Arthritis Mutilans.

Kate killebrew[11] found higher incidence of new bone formation i.e.82% of 87 study cases. Avila et al[7] had exactly the same incidence of erosions in 23%of 150 study cases.

Martel et al[13] had reported a slightly higher incidence of erosions i.e.30% of 50 study cases.

Peterson et al[9] reported almost similar incidence of tuft resorption in 22% of 39 study cases, whereas Martel et al[13] got slightly higher results of 30% of 50 study cases.

Avila et al[7] found a higher incidence of mild flexion deformity and loss of articular cartilage in 16% each in 150 study cases.

Baker et al[8] also observed bony ankylosis in 3%of 60 study cases whereas Peterson et al[9] noticed much higher incidence of 15% of 39 study cases.

DISTRIBUTION OF RADIOLOGICAL FEATURES IN DORSOLUMBAR SPINE

The association of spondylitis was first observed by Zellner in 1928. In our study, psoriatic spondylitis was observed in 10(33%) of cases. The syndesmophytes in our study were coarse, non-marginal floating and unilateral in nature (Figure.9).

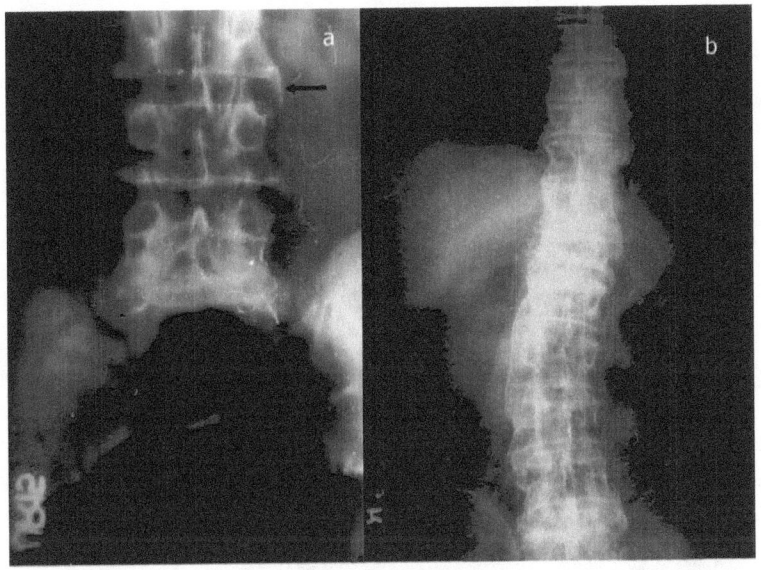

Figure.9 -(a)X ray lumbar spine AP view showing non marginal asymmetrical floating osteophytes arising from the bodies of L4 and L5 vertebrae(black arrows)(b)X ray dorsolumbar spine AP view showing coarse non marginal asymmetrical syndesmophytes involving L1-2,L2-3,L3-4 and L4-5 vertebrae on right side. Left side is spared. Note disc spaces are preserved.

Kate killebrew[11] noticed much higher incidence of syndesmophytes i.e. 68% of 87 study cases as compared to our study.

DISTRIBUTION OF RADIOLOGICAL FEATURES IN SACROILIAC JOINTS

In our study, the incidence of involvement of sacroiliac joints was in 10(33%) cases. The differ findings observed were articular erosions in 7(23%) cases, juxta articular sclerosis in 5(16.5%) cases and bony ankylosis in 2(6.6%) cases (Figure.10).

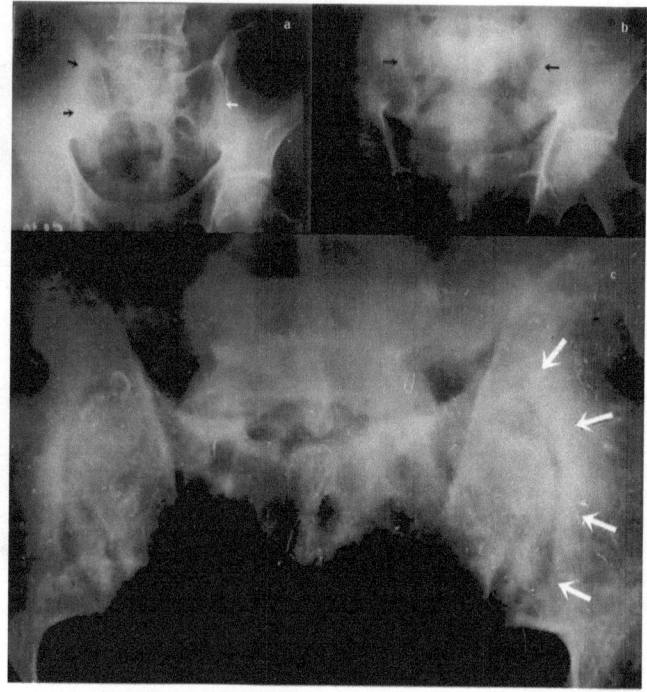

Figure.10-X ray both sacroiliac joints AP views (a)showing bony ankylosis right SI joint(black arrow),left SI joint is normal(white arrow) (b) Bony ankylosis of both SI joints -black arrows,(c) showing erosions in left SI joint with juxta articular sclerosis (white arrows).Right SI joint is normal(Asymmetric Sacroiliitis).

Peterson et al[9] has also reported similar incidence of sacroiliac joint involvement in 365 of 39 study cases. Baker et al[8] also reported similar results of articular erosions i.e.25% of 60 study cases.

Kate Killebrew et al[11] has observed slightly higher incidence of bony ankylosis i.e. 9% of 87 study cases.

Marsal et al[18] reported involvement of SI joint in 28% of 73 study cases, which has incidence nearly similar to our study.

D Kane et al[23] reported sacroiliitis in 17% of 129 study cases, which is less than that in our study.

CHAPTER V

SUMMARY

The present study was undertaken to determine radiologically various skeletal changes in clinically diagnosed cases of psoriasis with arthritis and to study the distribution pattern of various skeletal changes seen in psoriasis associated with commonly involved joints. Thirty psoriatic cases with arthritis that were seronegative for rheumatoid factor were enrolled. The observations were as follow:

Out of 30 study cases, 19(63%) were male and 11(37%) were females with male to female ratio 1.72:1. The mean age was 49 years with age range from 28-70 years. Maximum no. of cases 26(86.8%) were between 31-60years. 5(16.5%) cases gave positive family history. ESR was raised in 26(85.5%) cases. 9 (30%) cases suffered from mild anemia.

Commonest clinical pattern of psoriasis was discoid psoriasis i.e. in 20(66%) cases. The clinical presentation of arthritis was in form of pain in 18(60%) cases. Associated nail changes were observed in 24(80%) cases.

The duration of skin lesions in 17(56.1%) cases was more than 5 years and range of duration of skin lesions was 3 months to 25 years.

The duration of bony involvement in 10(33%) cases was between 6 months to 2 years and the age range of duration of bony involvement was 3 months to 20 years. In 21(80%) cases skin lesions preceded arthritis while in 6(20%) skin lesions started concomitantly with arthritis.

The commonest bony involvement observed in hands in 21(70%) cases, followed by feet in 19(63.3%) cases. Sacroiliac joint and dorsolumbar spine were involved in 10(33%) cases each. Hands, feet, SI joints and DL spine were involved in 4(13.2%) cases.

The most common radiological changes seen in hands was bare area erosions at distal interphalangeal joints in 21(70%) cases. Most common findings in feet were new bone formation at base of terminal phalanx of great toe in 19(63.4%) cases. The only radiological finding in dorsolumbar spine was coarse, asymmetrical, syndesmophyte in 10(33%) cases. Most common radiological finding in sacroiliac joints was articular erosions in 7(23%) cases.

Other radiological findings observed in hands and feet were tuft resorption, loss of articular cartilage, mild flexion deformity and bony ankylosis.

CONCLUSIONS

After reviewing the literature and in the light of aforesaid findings in the present study, it can be concluded that psoriatic arthritis definitely shows wide range of radiological skeletal changes. The most commonly sites involved are bare area erosions of distal interphalangeal joints of fingers and interphalangeal joints of great toe. The most common radiological findings are erosion in hands and new bone formation in feet. In spine dorsolumbar region is commonly involved in form of coarse, asymmetrical syndemophytes. Articular erosions is a common findings in sacroiliac joints.

COMMENTS

In routine, radiological assessment is not done in psoriatic cases with or without arthritis. We are of the opinion that every patient of psoriasis must be subjected to radiological examination so as:-

1. To detect arthritis at an early stage.

2. To start very early more aggressive therapy which might include methotrexate? rather than NSAIDs.

3. To stop the progression of joint destruction and disability.

4. To reduce gross deformities.

5. To limit the number of swollen, tender joints.

REFERENCES

1. Garrod and Geoffrey E. Arthropathica psoriatica by Archiablade. Quar Jour Med 1924:171-76.

2. McKenna RMB.Psoriatic arthritis.BMJ 1950; 2:207.

3. Sherman MS.Psoriatic arthritis.JBJS 1952;34A:831-52.

4. Eisenstadt HB,Arthur port.Arthritis Mutilans.1955;JBJS;37(2):337-46.

5. Wright V.Psoriasis and arthritis.BJD 1957; 69:628-33.

6. Wright V.Rheumatism and psoriasis.AJM 1959:454-62.

7. Avila Pugh DG,Winkelmann RK.Psoriatic arthritis. Radiology 1960; 75:691-701.

8. Baker H.Psoriasis and polyarthritis.BMJ 1963:348-52.

9. Peterson CC,Silbiger ML.Psoriatic arthritis.BJR.1967;(4):866-71.

10. Miller JL,Soltani K.Psoriatic acro-osteolysis;a case study. JBJS 1971;53(2):371-73.

11. Killebrew K,Gold RH,Sholkoff SD.Psoriatic spondylitis. Diagnostic Radiology 1973;108:9-16.

12. Schumacher E, Genant HK, Kellet MJ.HLA-B27 associated arthro pathies.Diagnostic Radiology 1978;126:289-97.

13. Martel W, Hylland RG. Erosive osteoarthritis and psoriatic arthritis. AJR.1980; 134:125-35.

14. Oriente S, Scarpa R, Pucino A. Prevelance of psoriatic arthritis in psoriatic patients. Acta Derm Vene 1984;113(suppl.):109-12.

15. Rajendra K, Madewell JE. Rheumatoid and seronegative arthropathies of foot. RCN.1987;25(6):1263-78.

16. El Khoury, Kathol MH, Brandser EA. Seronegative sponyloarthro pathies. RSNA 1996;34(2):343-57.

17. M Backhaus, T Kamradt, D Sandrock, D Loreck, J Fritz, KJ Wolf, H Raber, B Hamm, GR Burmester, M Bollow. Arthritis of the finger joints. Arthritis & Rheumatism 1999;42 (6):1232-45.

18. Marsal S, L Armadans Gil, M Martinez, D Gallardo, A Ribera, E Lience. Clinical, radiographic and HLA associations as markers for different patterns of psoriatic arthritis. Rheumatology 1999; 38; 332-37.

19. Brockbank J, Gladman D. Diagnosis and management of psoriatic arthritis. Drugs 2002;62(17):2447-57.

20. DD Gladman, C Antoni, P Mease, D O Clegg, P Nash. Psoriatic arthritis: epidemiology, clinical features, course, and outcome. Ann Rheum Dis 2005;64(Suppl II):ii14–ii17.

21. P A Ory,D D Gladman,P J Mease. Psoriatic arthritis and imaging.Ann Rheum Dis 2005;64(Suppl II):55–57.

22. CP Rajendran,SG Ledge,Kanaka P Rani,Radha Madhavan.Psoriatic Arthritis.JAPI 2003;51:1065-68.

23. D Kane,L Stafford,B Bresnihan,O Fitzgerald.A prospective, clinical, radiological study of early psoriatic arthritis;an early synovitis clinic experience.Rheumatology 2003; 42:1460- 68.

24. JE Brockbank,M Stein, CT Schentag,D D Gladman.Dactylitis in psoriatic arthritis: a marker for disease severity? Ann Rheum Dis 2005;64:188-190.

25. Camp RDR. Text book of dermatology(by rook).Psoriatic arthritis. Edi-92:1440-46.

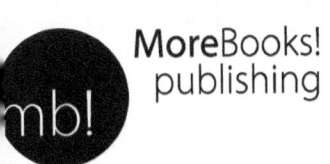
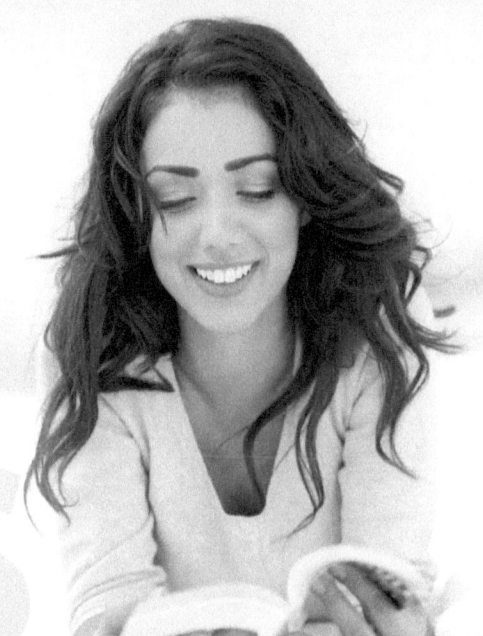

i want morebooks!

Buy your books fast and straightforward online - at one of world's fastest growing online book stores! Environmentally sound due to Print-on-Demand technologies.

Buy your books online at

www.get-morebooks.com

Kaufen Sie Ihre Bücher schnell und unkompliziert online – auf einer der am schnellsten wachsenden Buchhandelsplattformen weltweit! Dank Print-On-Demand umwelt- und ressourcenschonend produziert.

Bücher schneller online kaufen

www.morebooks.de

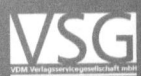 VDM Verlagsservicegesellschaft mbH
Heinrich-Böcking-Str. 6-8   Telefon: +49 681 3720 174   info@vdm-vsg.de
D - 66121 Saarbrücken   Telefax: +49 681 3720 1749   www.vdm-vsg.de

www.ingramcontent.com/pod-product-compliance
Lightning Source LLC
Chambersburg PA
CBHW031551210526
45464CB00003B/1248